Noom Diet
Cookbook And Meal Plan

Your Essential Guide to Effortless Weight Loss and
Lifelong Wellness

Anne Finley

TABLE OF CONTENTS

INTRODUCTION

Welcome to the Noom Diet, a novel approach to weight loss and good life. We urge you to embark on a revolutionary journey in this groundbreaking book, "Noom Diet Cookbook and Meal Plan," that will not only change your body but also transform your relationship with food.

Are you sick of diets that promise rapid cures but leave you feeling dissatisfied and defeated? The Noom Diet is a pleasant alternative to standard weight loss plans since it focuses on your physical, mental, and emotional well-being. It's time to abandon restrictive diets in favor of a sustainable lifestyle that delivers joy, balance, and long-term results.

A simple yet powerful principle sits at the foundation of the Noom Diet philosophy: understanding the psychology behind your eating patterns. Unlike other diets that focus exclusively on calorie monitoring or the elimination of specific food groups, the Noom Diet takes a personalized approach that is suited to your specific needs and tastes. This strategy helps you make thoughtful decisions, form healthy habits, and develop a positive connection with food by leveraging the power of behavioral psychology.

We will walk you through every stage of your Noom Diet journey in this detailed guide. We cover everything from learning the fundamentals of the Noom Diet to creating a balanced plate and stocking your kitchen with necessary items. You'll learn that eating properly doesn't have to mean compromising flavor or enjoyment with our collection of delectable and nutrient-dense dishes. Say goodbye to dull and uninteresting meals; we have a plethora of tempting selections for breakfast, lunch, supper, snacks, and even desserts.

But the Noom Diet is about more than just what you consume. We recognize that long-term weight loss and good living necessitate a multifaceted strategy. That is why we offer you important advice on creating goals, remaining motivated, and conquering obstacles. Our 14-day Noom Diet meal plan is intended to help you get started and give you structure while also promoting flexibility and personalization to fit your lifestyle.We provide you with the skills to maintain your healthy behaviors after the initial 14-day plan. We dig into the art of mindful eating, helping you to make a deeper connection with your body's signals and cultivating gratitude for the food it gets. We provide skills for navigating social situations, overcoming plateaus, and developing a healthy relationship with food that goes beyond the limits of a certain diet plan.

"Noom Diet Cookbook and Meal Plan" is your trusty companion, whether you're just starting your weight reduction journey or seeking a new strategy to maintain a healthy lifestyle. Allow us to assist you in embracing a sustainable way of eating that feeds your body, delights your taste buds, and takes you closer to the vibrant, confident version of yourself that you've always desired. Prepare for a voyage of self-discovery, gastronomic exploration, and transformational change. Join the Noom Diet movement today and say hello to a new you. Your body, mind, and taste buds will be grateful.

CHAPTER ONE

THE NOOM DIET: A REVOLUTIONARY APPROACH TO WEIGHT LOSS AND HEALTHY LIVING

Understanding the Noom Diet Philosophy

The Noom Diet concept is based on the idea that long-term weight loss and good living cannot be achieved by quick cures or harsh limitations. Instead, it takes a more comprehensive approach that focuses on the psychological, emotional, and behavioral elements of eating. The Noom Diet attempts to produce a lifetime shift in our connection with food and our bodies by recognizing the underlying causes that drive our eating choices and adopting healthy habits.

The Noom Diet, unlike typical diets that depend primarily on calorie monitoring or tight meal planning, understands the significance of treating the psychological issues that contribute to overeating and harmful behaviors. It uses the power of behavioral psychology to help people make more conscious decisions and establish a healthy relationship with food.

The Noom Color System is a crucial component of the Noom Diet. This approach divides foods into three color groupings depending on their calorie density and nutritional value: green, yellow, and red. Green vegetables are abundant in nutrients and low in calories, making them great for including in your regular diet. Yellow foods have a low calorie density and should be eaten in moderation. Red foods have more calories and should be taken in moderation.

The Noom Diet stresses portion management and encourages people to use the Noom Color System to produce balanced meals. Individuals may ensure that their meals are nutrient-dense and delicious while keeping calorie consumption in line by including a range of colorful foods from the green group. This method encourages a balanced and sustainable style of eating, ensuring that individuals get the nutrients they need while efficiently regulating their weight.

The emphasis on self-awareness and mindful eating is another important part of the Noom Diet concept. Individuals may gain a deeper awareness of their body's demands and make deliberate decisions about what and how much they eat by paying attention to hunger and fullness signs. Mindful eating means savoring each meal, being present in the moment, and paying attention to the body's hunger and satiety signals. Individuals may make more informed decisions and build a healthy connection with food by gaining this knowledge.

Furthermore, the Noom Diet understands that long-term success is not exclusively determined by what happens at the dinner table. It recognizes the influence of external influences on our eating behaviors, such as social contexts, emotional triggers, and stress. The Noom Diet concept gives tools and tactics to help people negotiate these hurdles, allowing them to make better choices even in tough situations.

How the Noom Diet Works

By combining psychology, nutrition, and behavior modification strategies, the Noom Diet offers a novel and successful approach to weight loss and good living. It is based on the premise that long-term success is obtained through consistent and deliberate adjustments in eating habits and lifestyle choices.

1. **Trained examination:** When you begin the Noom Diet, you are subjected to a tailored examination procedure. This entails responding to questions about your existing way of life, aspirations, preferences, and obstacles. This examination

assists in developing a customized strategy that meets your individual needs and lays the groundwork for your trip.

2. Behavioral Change approaches: To address the psychological components of eating, the Noom Diet combines behavioral change approaches. Noom assists you in identifying and changing thinking patterns, emotions, and behaviors that lead to harmful eating habits through cognitive behavioral therapy (CBT) and other evidence-based approaches. You may create healthier relationships with food and make more conscious decisions if you understand the triggers, habits, and emotional connections to food.

3. The Noom Color System divides meals into three categories: green, yellow, and red. This approach supports balanced eating by providing simple and visual guidance for portion control. Green foods, such as fruits, vegetables, and whole grains, are low in calorie density and abundant in nutrients. Yellow foods should be taken in moderation, such as lean meats and starchy vegetables. Red foods, particularly higher-calorie products like candies and processed snacks, should be consumed in moderation. The Color System assists you in making educated food choices and encourages a well-balanced, nutrient-dense diet.

4. Calorie Tracking and Monitoring: Noom includes easy-to-use software for tracking your daily food consumption, activity, and progress. Logging your meals and activities helps you become aware of your calorie consumption and allows you to make modifications as needed. The app gives feedback and nutritional information and assists you in staying on track with your goals.

5. Support and Guidance: Noom offers continuing assistance via a virtual community and a personal health coach. You may connect with others on the same road, exchange experiences, and seek encouragement in the community. Furthermore, your personal health coach provides direction, accountability, and aid in overcoming obstacles.

6. Mindfulness and Education: The Noom Diet goes beyond calorie tracking by providing educational tools to help you better understand nutrition, portion sizes, and good eating habits. You'll discover the nutritional value of foods, how to find better replacements, and how to incorporate mindful eating habits into your everyday routine. You may create a healthy connection with food and make more mindful decisions by being more aware of your body's hunger and fullness cues.

7. Long-term Sustainability: The Noom Diet is intended to be a long-term solution, not a quick fix. It promotes slow and consistent weight reduction with the goal of losing 1-2 pounds each week, which is considered a healthy and manageable rate. The Noom Diet helps you maintain healthy behaviors after the first weight reduction phase by concentrating on behavior modification, mindfulness, and education.

Benefits of the Noom Diet

As a certified dietitian, I can detail various possible Noom Diet advantages. Individual results may vary, so it's best to talk with a healthcare expert before embarking on any new diet or weight reduction program. Here are some of the Noom Diet's possible advantages:

1. Lasting Weight Loss: The Noom Diet focuses on slow and lasting weight loss, with a weekly goal of 1-2 pounds. This strategy encourages practical and lasting lifestyle adjustments rather than severe and unsustainable methods, which promotes long-term success.

2. Mindful Eating and Behavioral Change: The Noom Diet integrates behavioral change strategies and supports mindful eating habits. Individuals may create healthier connections with food, increase portion management, and make more conscious decisions by addressing the psychological components of eating and boosting awareness of hunger and fullness cues.

3. Holistic Approach to Health: The Noom Diet approaches health holistically, taking into account not just diet but also psychological, emotional, and lifestyle elements. Individuals may enhance their overall well-being and develop long-term healthy behaviors by addressing these distinct components.

4. Nutrient-Dense Meals: The Noom Color System promotes nutrient-dense meals such as fruits, vegetables, whole grains, and lean meats. These foods supply critical vitamins, minerals, fiber, and other nutrients required for good health. Individuals may improve their general nutrition and well-being by concentrating on nutrient-dense foods.

5. Community Support and Personal Coaching: Noom offers a virtual community as well as a personal health coach to provide support, direction, and accountability.

Individuals may use the community to connect with others on the same road, exchange experiences, and seek encouragement. Personal health coaches offer specialized advice, answer concerns, and assist clients in overcoming obstacles, all while encouraging a sense of support and inspiration throughout the process.

6. Empowerment and Education: The Noom Diet provides instructional materials to help people better understand nutrition, portion sizes, and good eating habits. The Noom Diet empowers individuals with knowledge and information, allowing them to make educated decisions, build better habits, and achieve long-term success.

7. Personalization and Flexibility: The Noom Diet understands that everyone's choices, lives, and demands are unique. It allows for customization and flexibility, allowing people to tailor the program to their own circumstances and goals. This adaptability can help people stick to their diet and make it a part of their lifestyle.

CHAPTER TWO

GETTING STARTED WITH THE NOOM DIET

Setting Goals and Creating a Personalized Plan

Setting objectives and developing a specific strategy are critical elements in succeeding with any diet or lifestyle change, including the Noom Diet. You can remain motivated, measure progress, and achieve long-term improvements by defining clear targets and personalizing a strategy to your individual requirements. Here's a discussion on goal setting and developing a tailored plan:

1. Identify Your unique Goals: Begin by determining your unique goals. Do you want to reduce weight, improve your general health, manage a specific health issue, or increase your level of fitness? Make it clear and detailed what you aim to achieve. Setting quantifiable and attainable objectives can assist you in remaining focused and motivated throughout your trip.

2. Evaluate Your Current Lifestyle: Examine your current dietary habits, physical activity level, and lifestyle aspects that may affect your health. Consider your job schedule, family obligations, and social activities. Understanding your starting point will enable you to discover areas for development and make necessary changes.

3. Divide Goals into Smaller Tasks: Instead of focusing entirely on the ultimate result, divide your goals into smaller, more doable tasks. This method prevents overload and allows you to appreciate your accomplishments along the way. Set monthly or weekly milestones that match your long-term goal, for example, if you want to lose weight.

4. Develop a Realistic Timeline: Consider the period in which you want to attain your objectives. Be realistic and accept that long-term transformation takes time. Avoid establishing unrealistic deadlines that may result in irritation or unsustainable behaviors. A slow and methodical approach is more likely to provide long-term outcomes.

5. Identify Specific Action Steps: Once you've identified your goals, figure out what steps you need to take to get there. These steps might include changing your eating habits, boosting your physical activity, adopting mindful practices, or addressing emotional food triggers. Divide your strategy into concrete stages that are both achievable and feasible for you.

6. Monitor and Track Your Progress: It is critical to regularly monitor and track your progress in order to stay accountable and inspired. Record your meals, activities, and milestones using tools such as food and exercise notebooks, smartphone applications, or wearable gadgets. This data will give you insights into your development and assist you in making necessary modifications.

7. Be Flexible and adaptable: Recognize that circumstances might change and that adaptability is essential for long-term success. If particular techniques or approaches aren't working for you, be willing to change your strategy. Consider hiring a personal health coach or joining a supportive group to help you negotiate obstacles and stay on track.

Understanding the Noom Color System

Understanding the Noom Color System is essential to the Noom Diet. This approach divides foods into three categories depending on their calorie density and nutritional value: green, yellow, and red. The Color System helps people make educated food choices and promotes healthy eating. Here's an explanation of each color type and its meaning:

1. Green Foods:

- Green foods have a low calorie density but a high nutritional value. They are thought to be the most nutrient-dense and health-promoting foods.

- Most fruits and vegetables, whole grains, legumes, nonfat dairy, and lean proteins are examples of green foods.

- These items are recommended and should form the basis of your meals. They provide important vitamins, minerals, fiber, and other healthy ingredients while being low in calories.

2. Yellow Foods:

- Yellow foods have a low-calorie density and should be eaten in moderation.

- Yellow foods include lean meats such as skinless poultry and fish, low-fat dairy products, whole grain bread, and starchy vegetables such as sweet potatoes and maize.

- Yellow foods are still healthy and have a role in a balanced diet, but they should be consumed in moderation to maintain calorie balance.

3. Red Foods:

- Red foods have a greater calorie density and should be taken in moderation.
- Sugary sweets, fried meals, processed snacks, fatty cuts of meat, and full-fat dairy products are examples of red foods.

Tracking Your Food and Exercise

Tracking your diet and activity is an important part of the Noom Diet and will help you reach your health and weight reduction objectives. You obtain useful insights into your behaviors, make educated decisions, and stay accountable by keeping a record of what you consume and tracking your physical activity. Here's an explanation of the significance and advantages of diet and activity tracking:

1. Increased Awareness: Keeping a diet and exercise journal will help you become more aware of your everyday behaviors and patterns. It emphasizes portion amounts, food types ingested, and the overall balance of your meals. This enhanced awareness enables you to discover areas for improvement, make more deliberate decisions, and build healthier eating habits.

2. Portion management: One of the key benefits of meal monitoring is the effect it has on portion management.

You can properly measure and track the amount of food you consume by documenting your meals. This knowledge allows you to better understand acceptable portion sizes and make necessary modifications to correspond with your goals.

3. Nutritional Insight: Keeping a meal diary gives useful nutritional information. You may examine the balance of macronutrients (carbohydrates, proteins, and fats) in your diet by keeping a food diary. This knowledge allows you to make changes and guarantee you're reaching your nutritional requirements.

4. Accountability: Tracking your meals and activities might help you stay on track. Knowing that you must keep track of your choices motivates you to make healthy choices and stick to your goals. It also aids in the identification of prospective areas for development and holds you accountable for your progress.

5. Behavior Change: Tracking helps you detect trends and triggers that may have an influence on your food and activity habits. Recognizing these patterns allows you to make intentional attempts to change behavior and establish healthy routines. For example, if you realize that you have a habit of mindlessly snacking in the evening, monitoring can assist you in identifying this behavior and devising alternate techniques to control it.

6. Motivation and improvement Tracking: Logging your meals and activities allows you to see your improvement over time. As you notice positive improvements and achievements, it might act as inspiration to continue on your health path. It allows you to keep track of your achievements, create new objectives, and celebrate your successes.

7. Identifying issue Areas: Keeping track of your meals and activities will assist you in identifying issue areas that may be impeding your development. It enables you to detect potential triggers, emotional eating behaviors, or poor food choices that are inhibiting your performance. With this knowledge, you can devise ways to address and overcome these obstacles.

8. Personalization and Adaptation: Tracking gives essential data that may be utilized to customize and adjust your plan. You can identify what works best for you, make modifications, and enhance your strategy by evaluating your diet and activity diary.

Overcoming Challenges and Staying Motivated

Overcoming obstacles and staying motivated are critical components of success in any health and wellness journey, including the Noom Diet. Here are some techniques to help you overcome obstacles and stay motivated:

1. Establish reasonable and Achievable objectives: Begin by establishing objectives that are both reasonable and reachable. Break them down into smaller goals and celebrate each one along the way. Setting unrealistic objectives might result in dissatisfaction and motivational loss. Remember that development takes time, and long-term changes are created gradually.

2. Discover Your "Why": Determine your underlying motivations for making health and lifestyle improvements. Understanding your reasons and connecting with your underlying beliefs will help you stay engaged and motivated. To keep focused on your goals, remind yourself of these reasons on a frequent basis.

3. Celebrate Non-Scale Victories: Move your emphasis away from the number on the scale. Recognize and appreciate non-scale accomplishments like higher energy, better sleep, increased strength, or improved happiness. Recognizing these accomplishments may improve your motivation and remind you of the benefits of your work.

4. Create a Support Network: Surround yourself with a network of people who understand and support your goals, such as family, friends, or others who share your interests. Share your experience with them, seek their help, and rely on them at difficult times. Engage with the Noom community for more support, or consider hiring a personal health coach.

5. Keep Track of Your Progress: Keeping track of your progress can help you stay motivated. Record your accomplishments, milestones, and good improvements in a notebook, a smartphone app, or a visual tool. Seeing how far you've come might give you a sense of success and motivate you to continue.

6. Embrace Positivity and Self-Compassion: Throughout your path, practice positive self-talk and self-compassion. Be gentle with yourself, recognize your efforts, and concentrate on the good parts of your advancement. A good mentality may help you overcome obstacles and stay motivated.

7. Learn from Mistakes: Mistakes and obstacles are an inevitable part of every journey. Consider them chances for development and learning rather than failures. Analyze what caused the setback, devise plans for improvement, and modify your approach as needed. Remember that failures do not determine your development; what counts is how you respond to them.

8. Seek variation and Enjoyment: In order to keep things interesting and minimize monotony, include variation in your food and workout programs. Discover new nutritious foods, experiment with new types of physical activity, and find fun ways to keep active. Finding delight in your path makes it simpler to stay motivated and devoted.

9. Practice Self-Care: Look after yourself outside of your food and activity objectives. Prioritize rest, relaxation, and enjoyable activities. To guarantee a well-rounded approach to your general well-being, engage in hobbies, use stress-management skills, and prioritize self-care.

10. Review and reassess your goals and plan on a frequent basis: Review and reassess your goals and plan on a frequent basis. This allows you to make changes, create new goals, and ensure that your objectives remain in line with your changing requirements and preferences. A dynamic and adjustable strategy can aid in long-term motivation.

CHAPTER THREE

BUILDING A BALANCED NOOM PLATE

The Importance of Portion Control

When it comes to obtaining and maintaining a healthy weight, as well as encouraging general well-being, the importance of portion management cannot be overemphasized. Portion management is essential for promoting balanced nutrition, avoiding overeating, and developing a better relationship with food. Here are a few of the main reasons why portion control is essential:

1. Calorie management: Portion management is critical for controlling calorie intake. Controlling portion sizes helps ensure that you consume the right number of calories for your body. Excess calorie consumption can result in weight gain and an increased risk of chronic illnesses such as obesity, diabetes, and heart disease. You may maintain a better energy balance by limiting your portion sizes.

2. Nutrient Balance: Portion control aids in the attainment of a well-balanced diet. It allows you to designate various food categories on your plate, ensuring that you eat a range of critical nutrients. You may increase your nutritional intake and promote optimal health by including adequate quantities of fruits, vegetables, whole grains, lean meats, and healthy fats.

3. Attentive Food Selections: Portion control improves attentive food selections. Paying attention to portion sizes makes you more aware of the nutritional value and quality of the meals you eat. It aids in the prevention of overeating on unhealthy, calorie-dense meals such as those heavy in added sugars, harmful fats, and refined carbs. Instead, you may prioritize nutrient-dense selections and make better educated choices about what and how much to consume.

4. Awareness of Hunger and Satiety: Portion management increases your awareness of hunger and satiety cues. You can identify and accept your body's natural signals of fullness and pleasure by practicing portion management. This reduces overeating and creates a better connection with food by teaching you to listen to your body's needs instead of depending on external cues or emotional triggers.

5. Weight Control: Portion control is an important part of weight control. You may create a caloric balance that supports weight reduction, weight maintenance, or progressive weight increase by ingesting proper portion sizes. Portion management aids in the prevention of excessive calorie consumption, which is a common contributor to weight gain. It enables you to make informed decisions regarding portion sizes and assures

6. Long-Term Sustainability: Developing portion management practices aids in the long-term achievement of a healthy weight and general well-being. It is a long-term strategy that promotes moderation and balance while allowing for flexibility and enjoyment. Portion management is adaptive to varied contexts and lifestyles since it may be used in a variety of settings, such as dining out, social events, and home-cooked meals.

7. Mindful Eating Practices: Portion control and mindful eating are inextricably related. When you pay attention to portion sizes, you become more present and conscious of the food you consume. This attentiveness improves your whole eating experience, promotes better enjoyment, and aids in the prevention of thoughtless overeating.

Selecting the Right Balance of Colors

Choosing the proper color balance from the Noom Color System is an important part of the Noom Diet. You can construct a well-balanced and nutritious eating plan by learning the different color groups and implementing them into your meals. Here's a guide to choosing the proper color balance:

1. Make Green Foods a Priority: Green foods, which are low in calorie density but rich in nutritional content, should be the cornerstone of your meals. Incorporate a range of green fruits, veggies, whole grains, and nonfat dairy products. These foods include important vitamins, minerals, fiber, and other useful ingredients while being low in calories. To guarantee a nutrient-dense and balanced diet, make green items a large component of your meal.

2. Yellow Foods in Moderation: Yellow foods with a moderate calorie density should be taken in moderation. Lean proteins such as skinless poultry, fish, low-fat dairy products, whole-grain bread, and some starchy vegetables such as sweet potatoes and maize are examples. While these meals are high in nutrients, it is critical to watch portion sizes to maintain a healthy calorie balance. To promote a well-rounded and fulfilling eating plan, include modest amounts of yellow foods in your meals.

3. Limit Red Foods: Red foods, which have a greater calorie density, should be consumed in moderation. Sugary sweets, fried meals, processed snacks, fatty cuts of meat, and full-fat dairy products are examples of red foods. Because of their increased calorie content, these foods should be consumed in moderation. To maintain a balanced and calorie-conscious approach, exercise portion control and consume red foods in moderation.

4. Make Colorful and Varied Meals: Aim for colorful and varied meals by including a variety of foods from each color category. This not only results in a more visually pleasing meal, but it also enhances the probability of absorbing a diverse range of critical nutrients. Incorporate a variety of colored fruits, veggies, nutritious grains, lean proteins, and dairy products into your meals. This strategy increases dietary variety and general wellness.

5. Emphasize entire Foods: Regardless of color category, if feasible, emphasize entire, unprocessed foods. Whole foods are higher in nutritional density and include a greater spectrum of vitamins, minerals, and other useful components. Choose healthy grains over refined grains, fresh fruits and vegetables over canned or processed varieties, and lean proteins with few extra additives. Incorporating whole meals ensures that you get the most nutritional value out of the things you eat.

6. Consider Meal Composition: When arranging your meals, strive for a color balance on your plate. Aim for a mix of green, yellow, and red foods that correspond to your nutritional objectives. A well-balanced lunch can consist of a colorful salad with a variety of leafy greens, lean protein, and a modest serving of whole grain bread, for example. You may establish a suitable balance of colors and nutrients by examining the content of your meals.

Creating Nutrient-Dense Meals

Certainly! Here are a few examples of nutrient-dense meals that use the Noom Color System to integrate a range of colors:

Grilled Salmon with Quinoa and Roasted Vegetables:

- Grilled salmon (lean protein, omega-3 fatty acids)
- Quinoa (whole grain, high in protein)
- Roasted broccoli, bell peppers, and sweet potatoes (green and yellow vegetables)
- Drizzle of olive oil and lemon juice (healthy fats)

2. Veggie Stir-Fry with Brown Rice:

- Tofu or lean chicken breast (protein)
- Stir-fried mixed vegetables such as bell peppers, carrots, snap peas, and mushrooms (green and yellow vegetables)

- Brown rice (whole grain)
- Stir-fry sauce made with low-sodium soy sauce, ginger, and garlic

3. Colorful Salad with Grilled Chicken:

- Mixed salad greens (green vegetables)
- Sliced grilled chicken breast (protein)
- Cherry tomatoes and cucumber slices (red and green vegetables)
- Sliced avocado (healthy fats)
- Sprinkle with nuts or seeds (for additional healthy fats and crunch).
- Balsamic vinaigrette dressing (moderation)

4. Omelette with Spinach and Feta Cheese:

- Eggs or egg whites (protein)
- Fresh spinach leaves (a green vegetable)
- Crumbled feta cheese (moderation, flavor)
- Sliced tomatoes (a red vegetable)
- Whole grain toast (whole grain)

5. Lentil and Vegetable Curry with Quinoa:

- Lentils (protein, fiber)
- Mixed vegetables like cauliflower, bell peppers, and carrots (green and yellow vegetables)

- Coconut milk (healthy fats, flavor)
- Curry spices (flavor)
- Serve over cooked quinoa (whole grain).

6. Greek Yogurt Parfait:

- Plain Greek yogurt (protein, calcium)
- Mixed berries (antioxidants)
- Chia seeds or nuts (healthy fats, fiber)
- Optional drizzle of honey or sprinkle of cinnamon (in moderation)

CHAPTER FOUR

NOOM DIET KITCHEN ESSENTIALS

Stocking Your Pantry for Success

Having the correct foods in your pantry is essential for success on your health and wellness journey. A well-stocked pantry means that you have a wide range of nutritional alternatives on hand, making it easier to make balanced meals and snacks. Here's how to properly stock your pantry for success:

1. Whole Grains: Include quinoa, brown rice, whole wheat pasta, oats, and whole grain bread in your diet. These provide fiber, vitamins, minerals, and long-lasting energy.

2. Legumes: Include legumes such as lentils, chickpeas, black beans, and kidney beans. They are high in protein, fiber, and other important nutrients and may be used in soups, stews, salads, and as a meat replacement.

3. Healthy Fats: Choose healthy fat sources such as olive oil, avocado oil, nuts, seeds, and nut butter. These fats promote satiety, supply necessary fatty acids, and promote general health.

4. Low-sodium canned products: Stock up on low-sodium canned goods such as chopped tomatoes, tomato sauce, and canned beans. They make an easy basis for many dishes, providing flavor and nutrition.

5. Herbs and Spices: Keep a variety of herbs and spices on hand to add flavor to your meals without depending on too much salt or harmful sauces. Basil, oregano, turmeric, cinnamon, paprika, and garlic powder are a few examples.

6. Condiments and Sauces: Choose low-sodium soy sauce, balsamic vinegar, mustard, salsa, and hot sauce as healthier condiments and sauces. These may bring taste and diversity to your meals while avoiding the use of excessive sweets or harmful chemicals.

7. Canned Fish: Keep canned tuna, salmon, and sardines on hand. These are high in omega-3 fatty acids and can be used in salads, sandwiches, or as a protein source in a variety of meals.

8. Dried Herbs and Vegetable Broth: Keep dried herbs like thyme, rosemary, and bay leaves on hand, as well as vegetable broth or bouillon cubes. These may be used to improve the flavor of your food and can be added to soups, stews, and sauces.

9. Nutritious Snacks: Keep a variety of healthy snacks on hand, such as unsalted almonds, seeds, dried fruits, and whole grain crackers. These alternatives to processed foods are filling and nutrient-dense.

10. Fresh Produce: While not stored in the pantry, be sure to stock up on fresh fruits and veggies on a regular basis. Choose a range of brightly colored foods to include in your meals and snacks.

11. Hydration Options: Keep hydrated by stocking up on water, herbal teas, and low-calorie flavored water. Avoid sugary beverages in favor of hydrated ones that do not include added sugars.

Essential Tools and Gadgets

The correct kitchen equipment and gadgets may make meal preparation and healthy cooking more efficient and pleasurable. Here are some crucial kitchen equipment and devices to help you succeed in the kitchen:

1. Chef's Knife: For slicing, dicing, and cutting fruits, vegetables, and meats, invest in a high-quality chef's knife. A sharp and dependable knife simplifies and protects food preparation.

2. Cutting Board: Select a durable cutting board made of materials such as bamboo or plastic. Cross-contamination may be avoided by using a separate cutting board for fruits and vegetables and another for raw meats.

3. Measuring Cups and Spoons: Precise measuring is essential for portion management and recipe execution. Having a measuring cup and spoon set guarantees that you can follow recipes accurately.

4. Food Scale: A digital food scale is an excellent tool for portion management, particularly when measuring items by weight. It allows you to more accurately measure and regulate your food consumption.

5. Nonstick Cookware: Purchase a nonstick frying pan and pots to avoid the need for additional oil or fat when cooking. They facilitate cleanup and encourage healthier cooking practices.

6. Baking Sheet: When roasting veggies, baking homemade granola, or producing healthier versions of baked goods, a baking sheet is important. For uniform heat distribution, use a high-quality nonstick baking sheet.

7. Blender or Food Processor: A blender or food processor is useful for making smoothies, sauces, dips, and homemade nut butters. It enables you to create nutritious and flavorful recipes with ease.

8. Steamer Basket: A steamer basket is a useful tool for preserving the nutrients in vegetables. Steaming helps preserve color, texture, and taste while reducing the need for additional fats.

9. Salad Spinner: A salad spinner aids in properly washing and drying leafy vegetables. It keeps your salads crisp and free of excess moisture, which makes them more delightful to consume.

10. Immersion Blender: Also known as a hand blender, an immersion blender is helpful for mixing soups, sauces, and smoothies right in the pot or container. It avoids the need for hot liquids to be transferred to a separate mixer.

11. Spiralizer: A spiralizer turns vegetables such as zucchini or sweet potatoes into noodle-like strands, making them a healthier alternative to traditional pasta. It adds diversity to your meals and encourages culinary creativity.

12. Slow Cooker or Instant Pot: These machines are useful for quickly making healthful one-pot meals. They enable batch cooking, tenderizing difficult chunks of meat, and cooking entire grains, beans, and soups quickly.

13. Storage Containers: Having a range of storage containers in various sizes aids in meal preparation and the storage of leftovers. Choose microwave-safe, leak-proof, and stackable containers.

Tips for Healthy Grocery Shopping

1. Plan Ahead: Make a weekly meal plan and a shopping list based on the meals you've scheduled. This allows you to focus and avoid making impulsive purchases of harmful items.

2. Shop the Perimeter: Fresh vegetables, lean meats, dairy goods, and whole grains are commonly found on the grocery store's outside aisles. To emphasize nutrient-dense foods, spend the majority of your shopping time in these categories.

3. Read and Understand Food Labels: Take the time to read and comprehend food labels. Look for items with few ingredients, few added sugars, little salt, and no trans fats. Take note of serving sizes and the nutritional value per serving.

4. Choose Whole Foods: Eat as many whole, unprocessed foods as possible. Fresh fruits and vegetables, whole grains, lean meats, and unprocessed dairy products are all good choices. These options are often more nutritional and have fewer added sweets, bad fats, and artificial chemicals.

5. Fill at least half of your supermarket cart with fruits and veggies. Aim to fill at least half of your grocery cart with a variety of fruits and vegetables. To guarantee a wide assortment of vitamins, minerals, and antioxidants, choose a variety of hues.

6. Choose Lean Proteins: Choose skinless poultry, fish, lean cuts of meat, tofu, tempeh, lentils, and low-fat dairy products as lean protein sources. These solutions supply important nutrients without a lot of saturated fat.

7. Incorporate Whole Grains: Choose whole grain alternatives such as brown rice, quinoa, whole wheat bread, and whole grain pasta. When compared to processed grains, these have more fiber, vitamins, and minerals.

8. Reduce Your Consumption of Processed and Sugary Meals: Reduce your consumption of highly processed meals, sugary snacks, sodas, and sweetened beverages. These foods are frequently heavy in added sugars, bad fats, and empty calories.

9. Be Aware of Portion Proportions: When shopping for things, especially packaged snacks and pre-processed meals, keep portion proportions in mind. To avoid overeating, use single-serve alternatives or divide larger items into reasonable quantities.

10. Shop on an Empty Stomach: Shopping on an empty stomach might lead to rash and unhealthy food selections. Eat a healthy supper or snack before going shopping to help you retain your self-control.

11. Remain Hydrated: Carry a water bottle with you while grocery shopping to remain hydrated. Thirst is frequently confused with hunger, resulting in the wasteful purchase of harmful foods.

12. Compare Prices and Brands: For more cost-effective and healthier alternatives, compare prices, read reviews, and investigate store brands. It is not always essential to purchase the most costly brands in order to obtain nutritional options.

13. Spend Less Time in Processed Food Aisles: Spend less time in aisles containing overly processed and unhealthy items like chips, cookies, and sugary cereals. Instead, look for whole foods in the outside aisles.

14. Practice Safe Food Handling: Inspect perishable foods for signs of deterioration or damage. Separate raw meats from other foods and keep them securely packed and refrigerated.

CHAPTER FIVE

BREAKFASTS TO FUEL YOUR DAY

Energizing Smoothies and Bowls

Energizing smoothies and bowls are an excellent way to provide your body with a surge of nutrients while also maintaining energy levels throughout the day. These delectable treats are high in vitamins, minerals, fiber, and antioxidants, making them ideal for a quick and healthy lunch or snack. Here's a talk on revitalizing smoothies and bowls, including their advantages and preparation tips:

Energizing Smoothies and Bowls Have the Following Advantages:

1. Energizing Smoothies and Bowls: Energizing smoothies and bowls are a wonderful way to cram a range of nutrient-dense items into a single serving. They frequently include a variety of fruits, vegetables, nuts, seeds, and superfoods, which provide a variety of vitamins, minerals, and antioxidants to enhance general health.

2. Quick and Convenient: Smoothies and bowls can be produced in a matter of minutes, making them an ideal choice for busy people looking for a quick and nutritious meal on the go. They require no cooking or preparation time and may be eaten as a grab-and-go option or at home.

3. Hydration Boost: Many energetic smoothies and bowls feature hydrating components with high water content, such as fruits and vegetables. This promotes appropriate hydration, which is necessary for sustaining energy levels, cognitive function, and general health.

4. Digestive Health: Smoothies and bowls frequently contain nutritional fiber-rich ingredients. Fiber improves digestion, increases satiety, and promotes gut health. Fiber-rich items such as fruits, vegetables, and chia seeds might help with digestion and general gut health.

5. Longevity: Energizing smoothies and bowls have a blend of carbs, protein, and healthy fats that work together to deliver long-lasting energy. They can help you feel content and concentrated throughout the day by stabilizing your blood sugar levels, preventing energy dumps, and keeping you feeling satiated and focused.

Tips for Creating Energizing Smoothies and Bowls:

1. Balance the ingridents: Include a variety of fruits, veggies, proteins, healthy fats, and optional superfood add-ins in your smoothies and bowls. This equilibrium ensures a wide range of nutrients and tastes.

2. Use Leafy Greens: To increase the nutritional value of your smoothies and bowls, add a handful of leafy greens such as spinach, kale, or Swiss chard. Vitamins, minerals, and fiber abound in leafy greens.

3. Include Protein: Include a protein source such as Greek yogurt, silken tofu, nut butter, or a scoop of protein powder. Protein keeps you full and promotes muscle repair and development.

4. Include Healthy Fats: To add healthy fats, add a tablespoon of nut butter, a handful of nuts or seeds, or a scoop of avocado. Fats aid in nutrition absorption and provide sustained energy.

5. Superfood Add-Ins: For an extra nutritious boost, consider adding superfood ingredients such as chia seeds, flaxseeds, hemp seeds, spirulina, or maca powder. These antioxidant-rich compounds have extra health advantages.

6. Liquid foundation: To attain the proper consistency, use a liquid foundation such as almond milk, coconut water, or plain water. Adjust the amount of liquid to your preferred thickness.

7. Customize the flavors: Experiment with different combinations of fruits, spices, and natural sweeteners like honey or dates to develop a taste profile that you enjoy. Spices such as cinnamon or ginger can improve the flavor and provide extra health benefits.

8. Toppings and Texture: Blend your ingredients until smooth, or leave some texture if desired. For added texture and aesthetic appeal, top your smoothies or bowls with more fruits, nuts, seeds, granola, or shredded coconut.

Hearty Omelets and Frittatas

Hearty omelets and frittatas are filling and healthy dishes that are ideal for breakfast, brunch, or a quick dinner. These meals are adaptable, allowing you to tailor the ingredients to your taste preferences and dietary requirements. Here's a description of robust omelets and frittatas, as well as some recommendations for making them:

Hearty Omelets and Frittatas: How to Make Them

1. Basic definition: An omelet is a meal formed by beating eggs and frying them on a pan, frequently with different ingredients wrapped inside. A frittata, on the other hand, is similar to an omelet but is normally cooked on the stovetop before being completed in the oven. It is prepared in a single, open-faced, round, or rectangular dish, making it easier to serve a larger group.

2. Versatility: Omelets and frittatas allow for limitless personalization. You may design a flavor profile that meets your tastes by combining items such as vegetables, cheese, cooked meats, herbs, and spices. They're a great way to use up leftover items and spice up your meals.

3. Nutrient-Dense: Omelets and frittatas are nutrient-dense foods because they contain protein-rich eggs, veggies, and occasionally cheese. Eggs provide high-quality protein, vitamins, and minerals, while veggies provide fiber, antioxidants, and a variety of micronutrients. You can make a well-rounded and satisfying supper by combining a variety of items.

 4. Satiety and Energy: The protein in omelets and frittatas promotes satiety and can help manage hunger throughout the day. This can help with weight management and keep you from overeating later in the day. These meals' combination of protein, healthy fats, and veggies also delivers lasting energy, making them an excellent choice for getting the day started correctly.

Tips for Making Filling Omelets and Frittatas:

1. Vegetables: To add flavor, texture, and nutrition to your omelets and frittatas, use a variety of veggies such as bell peppers, onions, spinach, mushrooms, and tomatoes. For extra protein, add cooked meats such as diced ham or turkey bacon.

2. Cheese Selection: For added taste, add a sprinkle of cheese to your omelets and frittatas. Depending on your taste preferences, choose from cheddar, feta, mozzarella, or goat cheese.

3. Herb and Spice Seasoning: Use herbs and spices to enhance the flavor of your omelets and frittatas. Fresh herbs such as parsley, basil, chives, or dill may offer a burst of flavor, and spices such as paprika, cumin, or black pepper can add depth and warmth.

4. Beat the Eggs: Before adding the eggs to the skillet, whisk them together until thoroughly blended. This promotes consistent texture and cooking throughout.

5. Nonstick Pan: To avoid the omelet or frittata from sticking and to facilitate easy flipping or sliding onto a dish, use a nonstick skillet or well-seasoned cast-iron pan.

6. Cooking Method: For omelets, cook one side until set before flipping or folding it over the contents. Frittatas are often prepared on the stovetop to firm the bottom and edges before being finished in the oven. This technique guarantees uniform cooking and a fluffy texture.

7. Garnish and serve: Once cooked, top your omelets and frittatas with fresh herbs, cheese, or a dollop of Greek yogurt. Serve hot or at room temperature, cut into wedges or squares. They can be eaten alone, with a side salad, or with whole grain bread.

Wholesome Granolas and Porridges

Wholesome granolas and porridges are healthy and comfortable breakfast alternatives that will get you started on the right foot. They are adaptable, allowing you to tailor the components to your taste preferences and nutritional requirements. Here's a discussion on healthy granolas and porridges, including their advantages and how to make them:

Explained Wholesome Granolas:

1. Basic definition: Granola is a morning cereal prepared from rolled oats, nuts, seeds, dried fruits, and sugars that is baked till crispy. It is frequently served with milk or yogurt, as a garnish for smoothie bowls, desserts, or as a snack.

2. Nutrient-Dense: Nutrient-dense granolas are made with whole grains. Rolled oats are high in fiber, vitamins, and minerals, whereas nuts and seeds are high in healthy fats, protein, and micronutrients. Dried fruits provide natural sweetness as well as fiber, vitamins, and antioxidants.

3. Flexibility: One of the advantages of granola is its adaptability. You may make it your own by adding your favorite nuts, seeds, and dried fruits or by changing the sweetness to your liking. It lets you experiment with tastes and make granola that meets your preferences and dietary needs.

4. Energy and Satiety: Granola's complex carbs, healthy fats, and protein deliver continuous energy and help you feel full throughout the morning. It can assist in maintaining a healthy blood sugar level by minimizing energy dumps and reducing mid-morning eating.

Explained Wholesome Porridges:

1. Basic definition: Porridge is a warming, soothing food cooked by cooking grains in water or milk, such as oats, rice, quinoa, or millet. It is an adaptable and healthy breakfast choice that can be modified with numerous toppings and flavorings.

2. Nutrient-Rich Grains: The grains used in porridge give important nutrients such as fiber, vitamins, minerals, and complex carbs. Whole grains are healthier than refined grains because they preserve the bran and germ, providing additional nutritional advantages.

3. Creamy and Comforting: Porridge has a creamy texture and may be served in a variety of ways, from thick and robust to smooth and creamy. It provides a pleasant and comfortable start to the day, especially during the winter months.

4. Toppings and Flavorings: Porridge can be flavored with fresh or dried fruits, nuts, seeds, spices such as cinnamon or nutmeg, honey, maple syrup, or a dab of nut butter. These ingredients provide more nutrients, tastes, and sensations.

Tips for Making Healthy Granolas and Porridges:

1. Keep Sweeteners Under Control: When creating granola or porridge, keep sweeteners under control. Instead of processed sugars, use natural sweeteners such as honey, maple syrup, or mashed bananas. Use them moderately to enhance sweetness without adding too much sugar.

2. Include Nuts and Seeds: For a nutritious boost, add a variety of nuts and seeds to your granola or porridge. Almonds, walnuts, chia seeds, flaxseeds, and pumpkin seeds are all high in healthy fats, protein, and critical elements.

3. Add Dried Fruits: For natural sweetness and a burst of flavor, add dried fruits like raisins, cranberries, or chopped dates to your granola or porridge. They also contribute fiber and antioxidants to the diet.

4. Experiment with Spices: Spice up your cereal or porridge by adding cinnamon, nutmeg, cardamom, or ginger. These spices bring warmth and richness to your morning meal.

5. Personalize Toppings: Add your favorite toppings to your granola or porridge. Fresh fruits, sliced bananas, berries, yogurt, nut butter, or granola can offer variety, texture, and nutrition.

6. Cook with Nut Milks or Plant-Based Milk: To add flavor and creaminess to your porridge, use almond milk, coconut milk, or other plant-based milks. These solutions are also appropriate for people who are lactose intolerant or live a vegan lifestyle.

CHAPTER SIX

SATISFYING LUNCHES AND LIGHT DINNERS

Flavorful Salads and Dressings

Salads and dressings with vivid tastes are an excellent way to add nutrient-rich foods and colorful flavors to your meals. Salads are diverse because they allow you to combine a range of fresh vegetables, fruits, proteins, and grains to make a filling and healthy dish. Dressings, on the other hand, add a burst of flavor to salads, improving their taste and enjoyment. Here's a description of tasty salads and dressings, as well as some methods for making them:

Salads with Lots of Flavor:

1. Nutrient-Dense: Salads are high in critical elements such as vitamins, minerals, fiber, and antioxidants. You may construct a nutrient-dense lunch that supports overall health and well-being by mixing a range of vegetables, fruits, proteins, and whole grains.

2. Customizable: Salads are very customizable, allowing you to personalize them to your taste preferences and nutritional requirements. You may mix and match ingredients, modifying ratios and portion sizes, to make a balanced and fulfilling salad.

3. Texture and Color: Flavorful salads have a variety of textures and hues, making them aesthetically appealing and delightful to consume. By combining various veggies, fruits, and garnishes, you can make a salad that is not only nutritional but also visually appealing.

4. Versatility: Salads can be served as a main meal, a side dish, or even as a light snack. They can be tailored to various nutritional needs, such as vegetarian, vegan, gluten-free, or low-carb alternatives.

Suggestions for Making Flavorful Salads:

1. Verity of greens: Start with a foundation of fresh leafy greens such as spinach, romaine lettuce, arugula, or mixed salad greens. These provide a nutrient-dense base for your salad.

2. Colorful veggies and Fruits: For extra nutrition and flavor, add a variety of colorful veggies and fruits to your salad. Cherry tomatoes, cucumbers, bell peppers, carrots, beets, berries, or citrus segments are some examples.

3. Protein Sources: Include a protein source to make your salad more full and fulfilling. Grilled chicken, salmon, tofu, chickpeas, boiled eggs, or quinoa are all options. Protein increases satiety and aids in muscle repair and development.

4. **Healthy Fats:** Include healthy fat sources such as avocado slices, almonds, seeds, or olives. These not only give taste but also vital fatty acids and contribute to a full sensation.

5. **Texture and crunch:** Toasted nuts, seeds, croutons, or crunchy vegetables like radishes or jicama may provide texture and crunch to your salad. This improves the whole dining experience.

6. **Fresh Herbs:** To add brightness and freshness to your salad, use fresh herbs such as basil, cilantro, mint, or parsley. Herbs contribute flavor and can improve the taste of the components.

Flavorful Dressings an Explanation

1. **Improve Flavor:** Dressings are used to improve the flavor of salads by combining tanginess, sweetness, creaminess, and spiciness. They have the ability to convert a plain salad into a tasty and memorable dinner.

2. **Personalization:** Dressings may be tailored to your tastes by modifying the amounts and types of ingredients

used. This allows you to make a dressing that matches the salad's contents.

3. Moisture and Balance: Dressings provide moisture to the salad, ensuring that every mouthful is well coated and tasty. They aid in the binding of the components, preventing a dry or tasteless salad.

4. Nutrients and Healthy Fats: Many dressings contain healthy fats from sources such as olive oil, avocado oil, or nut oils. These fats promote satiety and aid in the absorption of fat-soluble vitamins from salad elements.

Recipes for Flavorful Dressings

1. Flavor Balance: In your dressing, aim for a balance of acidity, sweetness, and saltiness. To obtain a harmonic flavor profile, combine lemon juice, vinegar (such as balsamic, apple cider, or red wine vinegar), honey, maple syrup, or soy sauce.

2. Use Healthy Oils: In your dressings, use healthier oils such as extra virgin olive oil, avocado oil, or sesame oil. These oils supply monounsaturated fats and give the dressing a rich and silky texture.

3. Fresh Ingredients: To add depth and freshness to your dressings, use fresh ingredients such as minced garlic, grated ginger, or finely chopped herbs. The flavor

60

and quality of the dressing are enhanced by the use of fresh ingredients.

4. Experiment with Flavors: Try different flavor combinations by adding ingredients like Dijon mustard, tahini, yogurt, citrus zest, spices, or even a dash of spicy sauce. This allows you to make one-of-a-kind dressings to suit your tastes.

Nourishing Soups and Stews

Soups and stews are filling and fulfilling meals that may deliver a variety of nutrients while also warming you from the inside out. They are adaptable recipes that can be made with a variety of ingredients, making them an excellent way to include vegetables, proteins, grains, and spices in your diet. Here's an explanation of healthy soups and stews, as well as some ideas for making them:

Explained Nourishing Soups and Stews:

1. Critical Nutrients: Soups and stews are great for getting a range of critical nutrients in one bowl. They frequently feature a combination of vegetables, proteins, and, on occasion, grains or legumes, all of which provide vitamins, minerals, fiber, and antioxidants to help with general health.

2. Hydration and Satiety: Because soups and stews are broth-based, they have a high water content. This helps you stay hydrated and can increase feelings of fullness and contentment. These meals' blend of liquids and ingredients might help you stay hydrated throughout the day.

3. Versatility: There are limitless ways to customize soups and stews. To fit your taste preferences and nutritional demands, you may experiment with different flavor profiles, spices, herbs, and ingredient combinations. There is a dish for everyone, whether you want a robust vegetable soup, a protein-packed chicken stew, or a plant-based chili.

4. Digestive Health: Soups and stews are frequently high in vegetables and fiber-rich components. This can help with digestion and produce regular bowel motions. The moderate heating method employed in soups and stews can also help break down vegetable fibers, making them simpler to digest.

Tips for Making Nutritious Soups and Stews

1. Broth or Base: As the foundation of your soup or stew, start with a tasty broth. Depending on your preferences and dietary requirements, you can use vegetable, chicken, beef, or bone broth. Homemade broth is preferable, although store-bought broth can still be used.

2. Vegetable Variety: Include a variety of veggies in your cuisine to offer color, texture, and nutrition. Carrots, celery, onions, bell peppers, tomatoes, sweet potatoes, leafy greens, and zucchini are among the examples. Experiment with seasonal produce to improve the flavor and nutritional profile.

3. Protein Sources: To make your soup or stew more filling, add proteins such as chicken, turkey, beef, tofu, tempeh, beans, lentils, or shellfish. Proteins aid in satiety and help the body repair and grow tissues.

4. Whole Grains or Legumes: To improve the fiber and nutrient content of your soup or stew, try adding whole grains like quinoa, barley, or brown rice, or legumes like chickpeas or lentils. These components provide prolonged energy and give the dish a hearty flavor.

5. Flavor Enhancers: To add depth and flavor to soups and stews, use herbs, spices, and seasonings. Garlic, ginger, turmeric, cumin, paprika, thyme, rosemary, and parsley are a few examples. As you proceed, taste and adjust the ingredients to your liking.

6. Simmering and Slow Cooking: To develop flavors and tenderize ingredients, let your soup or stew simmer or cook gently over low heat. This enables the flavors to blend, making a rich and tasty meal.

7. Quantity Cooking and Freezing: Soups and stews frequently taste better the next day, so make a larger quantity and freeze leftovers for future meals. They may be frozen in individual pieces for later use as quick and easy dinners.

8. Garnish and Serve: To improve the beauty and flavor of your soup or stew, consider adding fresh herbs, a squeeze of citrus juice, a dollop of yogurt or sour cream, a sprinkle of grated cheese, or a drizzle of olive oil before serving.

Creative Sandwiches and Wraps

Sandwiches and wraps are a creative and diverse way to have a great and balanced lunch. They let you layer different foods, textures, and flavors between two slices of bread or wrap them in a tortilla. Whether you like a traditional deli sandwich or a more daring fusion wrap, these masterpieces may be tailored to your tastes and dietary requirements. Here's a description of unique sandwiches and wraps, as well as some techniques for making them:

Sandwiches and Wraps Explanation:

1. Versatility: Creative sandwiches and wraps allow for unlimited customization. To make a unique and delectable mixture, mix and match ingredients: proteins, spreads, veggies, and sauces. This adaptability allows you to customize sandwiches and wraps to meet a variety of dietary preferences and constraints.

2. Nutritional Balance: Sandwiches and wraps can be made to create a well-rounded and balanced lunch. For satiety and muscle restoration, include proteins such as grilled chicken, turkey, tofu, or deli meats. For fiber, vitamins, and minerals, include a variety of veggies. For complex carbs, use whole grain bread or tortillas and incorporate healthy fats from spreads, avocado, or nuts.

3. Portability and Convenience: Sandwiches and wraps are easily portable, making them a practical alternative for on-the-go lunches. They may be prepared ahead of time and packed for work, school, picnics, or road vacations. Their portable nature removes the need for utensils, making them a convenient lunch alternative.

4. Texture and Flavor Variety: Creative sandwiches and wraps offer a variety of textures and flavors. You may incorporate crunchy components like lettuce, cucumbers, or toasted almonds, as well as creamy elements like spreads, cheese, or avocado. You may also experiment with other spices, herbs, or sauces to improve the flavor and make each mouthful fascinating.

Tips for Making Unique Sandwiches and Wraps:

1. Tortilla or bread selection: Select your base carefully. To improve the fiber and nutritional content of your sandwich or wrap, choose whole grain bread, bagels, pita pockets, or wraps. If you have certain dietary requirements, look into gluten-free or low-carb options.

2. Protein Options: Choose your protein source depending on your tastes and nutritional needs. Sliced turkey, roast beef, chicken, tuna, salmon, eggs, tofu, or tempeh are some of the alternatives. For increased diversity and flavor, blend various proteins.

3. Flavorful Spreads and Condiments: Add moisture and flavor to your sandwich or wrap with spreads and condiments. Consider mustard, hummus, pesto, Greek yogurt, salsa, tzatziki, or aioli as condiments. These can complement the other components and add a unique flavor.

4. Vegetable Medley: Add a variety of veggies to your sandwich or wrap for crunch, freshness, and nutritional value. Choose lettuce, spinach, tomatoes, cucumbers, bell peppers, sprouts, shredded carrots, or pickles. Don't be afraid to experiment with roasted or marinated veggies to enhance their depth of flavor.

5. Cheese and Extras: If you like cheese, add a piece or sprinkle of your favorite flavor. Extras such as sliced olives, sun-dried tomatoes, jalapeos, or caramelized onions may lend a layer of flavor and individuality to your dish.

6. Wrapping skills: If you're preparing a wrap, master basic wrapping skills to keep everything secure and minimize spillage. For easy handling, fold in the sides, roll firmly, and seal using toothpicks, or wrap in parchment or foil.

7. Pairings and Side Dishes: To make a balanced lunch, serve your sandwich or wrap with complimentary side dishes such as a side salad, vegetable sticks, baked chips, soup, or a fruit salad.

CHAPTER SEVEN

WHOLESOME MAIN COURSE MEALS

Colorful Vegetable Stir-Fries

Colorful vegetable stir-fries are not only visually beautiful, but also a healthful and savory way to consume a variety of veggies in one meal. Cooking bite-sized vegetables over high heat results in crisp yet soft vegetables that keep their brilliant colors and natural tastes. Here's a discussion of colorful vegetable stir-fries, including their advantages and preparation tips:

Colorful Vegetable Stir-Fries - How to Make Them:

1. Nutritious: Colorful vegetable stir-fries are high in vitamins, minerals, fiber, and antioxidants. Because different colored veggies contain different nutrients, eating a variety of colors offers a wide range of health advantages. Orange and yellow veggies, such as carrots and bell peppers, are high in vitamin A, whereas green vegetables, such as broccoli and kale, are high in vitamins C and K.

2. Balanced and Low-Calorie: Vegetable stir-fries may be a filling and low-calorie supper. They are often low in fat and high in fiber, which helps to keep you full and happy without consuming too many calories. You may boost the nutritional profile and satiety of the meal by adding lean proteins like tofu, chicken, or shrimp.

3. Convenient and quick: Stir-frying is a quick and easy cooking method that keeps the original tastes and textures of the veggies. You can have a wonderful and colorful lunch on the table in minutes by following a few easy steps. It's an excellent choice for busy people or those looking for a quick and nutritious meal.

4. Versatility: Vegetable stir-fries are quite versatile. You may use whatever mix of veggies you want or have on hand, making it simple to tailor the recipe to your tastes. This adaptability enables you to take advantage of seasonal food or use up leftover vegetables in your fridge.

How to Make Colorful Vegetable Stir-Fries:

1. Vegetable Selection: To make an eye-catching and healthful stir-fry, choose a range of vegetables with distinct colors, textures, and tastes. Bell peppers, broccoli, carrots, snap peas, mushrooms, zucchini, baby corn, bok choy, and snow peas are among examples. Feel free to investigate more choices based on your interests.

2. Vegetable Preparation: To achieve consistent cooking, wash and slice the veggies into similar-sized pieces. Some vegetables, such as broccoli and cauliflower, may benefit from blanching or steaming for a few minutes before stir-frying to ensure they are cooked through while still crisp.

3. Aromatics and Seasonings: Heat oil in a wok or big pan, then add aromatics such as garlic, ginger, or shallots to flavor the oil. Seasonings such as soy sauce, oyster sauce, hoisin sauce, or chili sauce can also be used to give depth and savory overtones. Experiment with different quantities to discover the appropriate balance for you.

4. Stir-Frying Technique: Stir-frying involves swiftly cooking veggies over high heat while stirring or tossing them constantly. This allows the heat to be distributed evenly and the veggies to be crisp-tender. It is important not to overcook them since brilliant colors and a small crunch are desired.

5. Timing: Begin by stir-frying heavier veggies, such as carrots or bell peppers, that require longer cooking periods. To avoid overcooking, add more delicate vegetables, such as snow peas or bean sprouts, at the end. This guarantees that the finished meal has a variety of textures and tastes.

6. Protein Option: For a balanced supper, add protein to your stir-fry. Thinly sliced chicken, beef, shrimp, tofu, or tempeh can be cooked alongside or separately from the veggies. Before serving, make sure the meats are well cooked.

7. Finishing Touches: Before serving, add extra flavor ingredients like sesame seeds, chopped fresh herbs like cilantro or Thai basil, or a drizzle of sesame oil. These garnishes add texture and boost the overall flavor of the stir-fry.

Lean Protein Delights

Lean protein treats are recipes that feature high-quality, low-fat protein sources. These recipes are not only tasty, but they also include crucial nutrients that promote satiety and help with muscle maintenance or growth. Lean proteins have less saturated fat and calories than their higher-fat cousins. Lean protein can help you maintain a healthy weight, improve your overall health, and satisfy your nutritional demands. Here's a summary of lean protein pleasures, including their advantages and various recipes:

The Advantages of Lean Protein:

1. Weight Control: Because lean proteins are frequently lower in calories and saturated fat, they are good for weight control. They give you a sensation of fullness and help reduce cravings, lowering your chances of overeating.

2. Muscle Repair and Growth: Protein is essential for muscle repair and maintenance. Lean protein consumption after exercise or during the day promotes muscle repair and development, especially when paired with regular resistance training.

3. Nutrient Density: Lean protein sources include a high concentration of vital elements such as vitamins, minerals, and amino acids. They are essential building blocks for many biological processes and promote general health and well-being.

Lean Protein Delights Examples:

1. Grilled Chicken Breast: A classic example of a lean protein treat is grilled chicken breast. It's low in fat, high in protein, and quite adaptable. It may be seasoned with herbs and spices, marinated, or used as a basis for salads, wraps, or stir-fries.

2. Fish: Lean protein and heart-healthy omega-3 fatty acids are abundant in fish such as salmon, tuna, trout, and cod. For a nutritious and filling lunch, serve grilled, roasted, or pan-seared fish with veggies or incorporate it into salads, tacos, or grain bowls.

3. Turkey: Turkey is a low-fat alternative to red meat. It comes in a variety of forms, such as ground turkey for burgers or meatballs, turkey cutlets for quick and easy dinners, and turkey breast for a lean protein centerpiece at holiday celebrations.

4. Legumes: Legumes, such as lentils, chickpeas, black beans, or kidney beans, are high in protein and fiber. They may be used as the major component in vegetarian cuisines such as lentil soups, chickpea curries, and bean salads, providing protein as well as plant-based nourishment.

5. Greek Yogurt: Greek yogurt is a protein-rich alternative that can be eaten on its own or used as a basis for smoothies, parfaits, or as a creamy topping for savory foods. It has less sugar and more protein than conventional yogurt, making it an excellent choice for adding lean protein to your diet.

6. Tofu and Tempeh: Tofu and tempeh are plant-based protein sources that are often used in vegetarian and vegan cooking. They absorb flavors well and may be stir-fried, roasted, or grilled to make excellent, protein-rich meals. They're also high in calcium and iron.

7. Egg Whites: Egg whites are a good source of lean protein. They may be made into omelets, scrambled eggs, or utilized in baking dishes. Egg white omelets with vegetables or a vegetable scramble are excellent ways to start the day with lean protein and nutrient-dense vegetables.

Grain and Legume-based Dishes

Grain and legume-based recipes are filling and diverse, including a variety of carbs, proteins, fiber, and other important elements. These recipes use grains such as rice, quinoa, barley, or bulgur, as well as legumes such as beans, lentils, or chickpeas. They can be served as main meals, sides, or as elements in salads, soups, and stews. Here's a review of grain- and legume-based foods, including their advantages and some popular recipes:

Grain- and legume-based dishes have the following advantages:

1. Nutrient Density: Grain and legume meals provide a variety of critical nutrients. Grains provide carbs, B vitamins, and minerals such as iron and magnesium. Legumes are high in plant-based proteins, fiber, folate, and other vitamins and minerals. They give a well-rounded nutritional profile when combined.

2. Plant-Based Proteins: Legumes are particularly beneficial since they are among the greatest plant-based protein sources. Combining legumes with grains results in a complementary protein supply that contains all of the necessary amino acids required by the body. As a result, grain- and legume-based recipes are excellent choices for vegetarians, vegans, and those trying to minimize their meat consumption.

3. Fiber Content: Fiber is abundant in grains and legumes. Fiber assists digestion, induces fullness, and aids in blood sugar regulation. Including grain- and legume-based meals in your diet can help your digestive system work properly and boost overall gut health.

4. Versatility: Grain- and legume-based recipes are extremely adaptable to a wide range of cultures and flavor characteristics. These recipes may be tailored to your taste preferences and culinary ingenuity, ranging from

Mediterranean grain salads to Indian lentil curries and Mexican bean burritos.

Grain and legume-based dish examples:

1. Rice and beans: Are a traditional combination found in many cuisines throughout the world. It goes well with a variety of spices and may be used as a filling for burritos, stuffed peppers, or as a side dish with grilled meats or vegetables.

2. Quinoa Salad: Quinoa is a protein-rich grain that may be used as the foundation for colorful and healthy salads. For a light and filling lunch, combine cooked quinoa with fresh veggies, herbs, and a zesty vinaigrette.

3. Lentil Soup: Lentils are adaptable legumes that cook rapidly. Lentil soups may be cooked with a variety of veggies, spices, and herbs to create a warm and comforting dish that's high in protein, fiber, and taste.

4. Chickpea Curry: Chickpeas, also known as garbanzo beans, are a popular legume used in a variety of dishes. Chickpea curry combines these protein-rich beans with spices, coconut milk, and veggies to create a tasty and healthy meal.

5. Barley Risotto: Barley is a chewy, nutty grain that may be used in place of rice in risotto recipes. It provides a creamy and pleasant meal when combined with veggies, herbs, and a tiny quantity of cheese.

6. Bulgur Salad: Bulgur is a whole grain derived from cracked wheat that is often used in Middle Eastern cuisine. It may be combined with colorful vegetables, herbs, and lemon juice to make a delicious and satisfying salad.

7. Black Bean Tacos: Black beans are a prominent legume in Mexican cuisine. Mash cooked black beans with seasonings and spread them into tortillas, then top with fresh veggies, salsa, and avocado for a wonderful plant-based taco alternative.

CHAPTER EIGHT

GUILT-FREE SNACKS AND APPETIZERS

Crispy Veggie Chips and Dips

Crispy vegetable chips and dips are a tasty and healthy alternative to typical potato chips and creamy dips. These chips are made from a variety of veggies and are finely sliced before being baked or air-fried till crispy, delivering a pleasing crunch. They may be coupled with a variety of tasty and healthful dips to complement the flavors and make a well-rounded snack or appetizer. Here's a description of crispy veggie chips and dips, as well as some techniques for making them:

Crispy Veggie Chips: How to Make Them

1. Nutrient-Dense: Because they are manufactured from a range of vegetables, veggie chips are a healthier alternative than normal potato chips. These chips provide vital vitamins, minerals, and dietary fiber that are found naturally in plants. They provide a convenient way to enjoy a snack while also introducing important elements into your diet.

2. Lower in Fat and Calories: Compared to standard potato chips, veggie chips are often lower in fat and calories. You may get a crispy texture without using excessive oil or bad fats by baking or air-frying thinly sliced veggies instead of deep-frying them.

3. Flavors and Textures: Veggie chips may be produced from a variety of vegetables, including root vegetables such as sweet potatoes, beets, or carrots, leafy greens such as kale or spinach, and even zucchini or parsnips. Each vegetable adds a distinct flavor and texture to the chips, providing a varied munching experience.

4. Homemade Alternative: Making your own veggie chips allows you to control the ingredients and tailor the tastes and spices to your desires. You may play around with different vegetable combinations and seasonings, making them a fun and creative culinary endeavor.

How to Make Crispy Veggie Chips:

1. Vegetable Selection: For superior chip texture, choose veggies that are firm and have a low water content. Sweet potatoes, beets, carrots, kale, zucchini, parsnips, or thinly sliced bell peppers are also popular options. To achieve equal cooking, slice them uniformly using a mandoline slicer or a sharp knife.

2. Vegetable Preparation: After slicing the veggies, wipe them dry to eliminate excess moisture and avoid crispiness. Toss them in a tiny quantity of olive oil or your favorite cooking oil, then season with your favorite spices or seasonings, such as sea salt, black pepper, garlic powder, paprika, or dried herbs.

3. Baking or Air-Frying: Arrange the seasoned vegetable slices on a baking sheet coated with parchment paper or in an air fryer in a single layer. Bake at a high temperature in a preheated oven or air fry until the chips are crispy and faintly golden brown. To avoid burning them, keep a tight watch on them.

4. Cooling and Storage: To obtain optimal crispiness, allow the vegetable chips to cool fully before serving. To keep their texture and flavor, store them in an airtight container. However, because there are no preservatives in homemade veggie chips, they may lose their crispiness with time, so eat them within a few days.

Dips for Crispy Veggie Chips: How to Make Them

1. Healthy Dip Alternatives: Combining crunchy vegetarian chips with healthy dips adds taste and improves the eating experience. Dips prepared from

Greek yogurt, hummus, salsa, guacamole, or bean-based spreads are high in protein, fiber, and minerals.

2. **Flavor Variations:** Dips may be tailored to your personal tastes. For a more strong flavor, try other ingredients and tastes, such as herbs, spices, lemon juice, or roasted garlic. Consider spinach and artichoke dip, roasted red pepper hummus, or avocado and lime salsa as appetizers.

3. **Nutritional Boost:** Dips prepared with Greek yogurt or bean-based spreads have more nutritional value than standard creamy dips. Greek yogurt is high in protein and calcium, but bean-based spreads are high in fiber, vitamins, and minerals. These healthier alternatives help to provide a more balanced snacking experience.

4. **Texture and Creaminess:** To complement the crunchy vegetable chips, dips should be creamy and smooth. To get the appropriate thickness, add a small amount of water or lemon juice.

Protein-packed Bites and Bars

Protein-packed bits and bars are quick and easy snacks that deliver a concentrated supply of protein as well as other important elements. These snacks are intended to help you achieve your protein requirements, induce satiety, and aid in muscle repair and development. Protein bites and bars come in a variety of flavors and variations, making them a simple and portable alternative for those on the move or as a post-workout snack. Here's an overview of protein-packed snacks and bars, as well as some advice for selecting or making them:

Protein-Rich Bites and Bars: An Overview

1. High-Quality Protein Source: Protein bites and bars are made using high-quality protein sources such as whey protein, casein protein, soy protein, or plant-based protein blends. These proteins contain amino acids that your body needs for a variety of purposes, including muscle repair and development.

2. Convenient and portable: Protein bites and bars are pre-packaged snacks that are readily portable, making them an ideal choice for individuals who lead hectic lives. They are portable and can be carried to work, the gym, or on the go, giving you a quick and simple intake of protein when you're on the go.

3. Satiety and Hunger Control: Protein has been shown to be more satiating than carbs or lipids. Including protein-packed nibbles and bars in your snack repertoire will help you reduce hunger, stay content between meals, and avoid overeating.

4. Muscle healing and Growth: Protein consumption after exercise is essential for muscle healing and growth. Protein-packed snacks and bars can help you restore your protein levels and assist muscle regeneration after exercise.

Choosing or Making Protein-Packed Bites and Bars:
1. Read the Nutrition Labels: When choosing protein bites and bars, read the nutrition labels to determine the protein content and protein sources. Choose items with at least 10 grams of protein per serving and a balanced macronutrient composition.

2. components: Read the ingredient list carefully and select snacks with high-quality protein sources, fewer added sugars, and natural components. Products with excessive levels of added sugars, artificial sweeteners, or harmful ingredients should be avoided.

3. Flavors and types: Protein bites and bars come in a variety of flavors and types to suit a variety of taste preferences and nutritional requirements. Experiment with several tastes to discover your preferences, whether they are chocolate, peanut butter, fruit, or nut-based.

4. Make Your Own Protein Bites: If you prefer homemade snacks, make your own protein bites with protein powder, nut butter, oats, nuts, and other items of your choosing. There are several recipes accessible online that allow you to tailor the flavors and textures to your preferences.

5. Portion Control: While protein bites and bars may be a nutritious snack, it's crucial to keep portion limits in mind. They can vary in size and calorie content, so read the serving size on the container and eat them in moderation to avoid consuming too many calories.

6. Personalize with Additions: If you like more texture and diversity in your protein bites or bars, consider adding other ingredients. Extra taste and nutrition can be added with chopped nuts, dried fruits, coconut flakes, or dark chocolate chips.

7. Consider dietary needs: Think about your nutritional demands. If you have certain dietary needs or limitations, seek out protein bits and bars that meet those needs. Individuals following vegetarian, vegan, gluten-free, or dairy-free diets have alternatives.

Savory and Sweet Snack Ideas

Snacks, both savory and sweet, offer a variety of alternatives for satisfying cravings and providing a nice pick-me-up throughout the day. There are lots of snack alternatives to fit your taste preferences, whether you want something salty and savory or something sweet and decadent. Here's a discussion of savory and sweet snack options, with examples from each:

Ideas for Savory Snacks:

1. Veggie Sticks with Hummus: Slice up fresh veggies like carrots, celery, bell peppers, or cucumber and serve with a tasty and protein-rich hummus dip.

2. Popcorn: For a low-calorie and fiber-rich snack, choose air-popped or lightly seasoned popcorn. To enhance flavor, sprinkle with herbs, nutritional yeast, or a little bit of your preferred seasoning.

3. Low-fat Cheese and Whole Grain Crackers: Pair a selection of low-fat cheeses or cheese sticks with whole grain crackers. This combo has a good amount of protein, fiber, and carbs.

4. Roasted Chickpeas: Drain and drain a can of chickpeas, mix with olive oil and spices, and bake until crispy. They make a tasty and protein-rich savory snack.

5. Mini Caprese Skewers: Thread on skewers cherry tomatoes, mozzarella balls, and fresh basil leaves. For a fast and tasty snack, drizzle them with balsamic glaze or season with salt and pepper.

6. Greek Yogurt with Herbs: Combine Greek yogurt with herbs such as dill, parsley, or chives for a creamy, protein-rich dip. Serve with whole wheat pita chips or veggie crudités.

Ideas for Snacks:

1. Fruit Salad: Make a pleasant fruit salad using seasonal fruits. This naturally sweet, nutrient-dense snack is high in vitamins, fiber, and antioxidants.

2. Yogurt Parfait: For a balanced and delightful sweet treat, layer Greek yogurt with fresh fruits, almonds, and oats. Choose plain Greek yogurt or one with little added sugar.

3. Dark Chocolate: Treat yourself to a square or two of high-quality dark chocolate with a cocoa level of 70% or more. Dark chocolate has a high antioxidant content and can fulfill your sweet desires.

4. Apple Slices with Nut Butter: Cut up apples and serve with a spoonful of natural nut butter, such as almond or peanut butter. Crisp apples and creamy nut butter make a tasty and wholesome combo.

5. Energy Balls: Combine nuts, seeds, dried fruits, and a touch of sweetness like honey or maple syrup to make homemade energy balls. These bite-sized sweets deliver an instant energy boost and may be tailored to your preferences.

6. Frozen Grapes: Freeze a bunch of grapes for a naturally sweet and refreshing snack. They have a pleasing texture and may be eaten right out of the freezer.

CHAPTER NINE

SWEET TREATS FOR DESSERT LOVERS

Noom-Approved Baked Goods

Noom advocates a whole-food, balanced approach to eating, with an emphasis on nutrient-dense foods. While there is no official list of "approved" baked goods, there are techniques to make healthier baked goods that adhere to Noom's values. Here are some Noom-friendly baking ideas:

1. Whole Grain Muffins: Make muffins with whole grain flours such as whole wheat or oat flour. For natural sweetness, add fruits such as bananas, apples, or berries. Reduce the amount of added sugar you consume or use natural sweeteners like honey or maple syrup instead. For extra texture and nutrients, try adding nuts, seeds, or shredded veggies.

2. Oatmeal Cookies: Use rolled oats as the major component in these cookies. Reduce the quantity of butter or oil used and replace it with natural sweeteners such as mashed bananas or applesauce. To add flavor and texture, mix with dried fruits, nuts, or dark chocolate chips.

3. Chia Seed Pudding: Make a tasty and nutrient-dense chia seed pudding. Chia seeds should be combined with unsweetened almond milk or Greek yogurt and a natural sweetener such as stevia or vanilla extract. Allow it to thicken in the refrigerator overnight. For extra crunch, top with fresh fruit or granola.

4. Sweet Potato Brownies: Use pureed sweet potatoes in place of part of the butter or oil in standard brownie recipes. Sweet potatoes contribute moisture and natural sweetness, as well as vitamins and fiber. For a deeper flavor, use dark chocolate or cocoa powder with a little additional sugar.

5. Protein Pancakes: Combine whole grain flour, protein powder, and mashed bananas or unsweetened applesauce to make pancakes. Avoid using additional sweeteners or syrups. To add flavor and nutrition, top with fresh fruits, yogurt, or a dab of natural nut butter.

6. Energy Bars: Make your own energy bars by combining nuts, seeds, dried fruits, and healthy grains such as oats. Avoid or limit the use of added sugars and syrups. Experiment with various flavors and textures by including spices such as cinnamon or cocoa powder.

Frozen Delights without the Guilt

Frozen treats may be enjoyed guilt-free by choosing healthier options that deliver wonderful tastes and pleasant textures while keeping nutritional value in mind. When compared to standard selections, these guilt-free frozen delights have fewer added sugars, harmful fats, and calories. Here's an explanation of guilt-free frozen treats, along with some examples:

1. Frozen Fruit Popsicles: Use pureed or blended fruits to make your own popsicles. Simply purée your favorite fruits, such as berries, mangoes, or watermelon, then pour into popsicle molds. If desired, add additional chopped fruits for texture. These handmade fruit popsicles are light, refreshing, and high in vitamins and fiber.

2. Greek Yogurt Parfait Popsicles: In popsicle molds, layer Greek yogurt and fresh fruits. Use plain or minimally sweetened Greek yogurt. The Greek yogurt adds nutrition and smoothness to the dish, while the fruits contribute natural sweetness and brilliant hues. This frozen delicacy provides nutritional balance as well as a pleasing flavor.

3. Banana "Nice" Cream: Freeze ripe banana slices. In a food processor or blender, puree the frozen banana slices until smooth and creamy. You may eat the banana "nice" cream alone or add a number of mix-ins such as chocolate powder, peanut butter, fruit, or almonds. This guilt-free dessert has the feel of ice cream without the extra sweets or dairy.

4. Frozen Yogurt Bites: Place spoonfuls of flavored Greek yogurt on a parchment-lined baking sheet and freeze until solid. These bite-sized delights have the creamy feel of frozen yogurt and may be personalized with additional fruits, nuts, or a drizzle of dark chocolate for more taste and texture.

5. Frozen Berries with Whipped Cream: Freeze a combination of fresh berries, such as strawberries, blueberries, or raspberries. Serve with a spoonful of unsweetened coconut cream or Greek yogurt whipped cream. Natural sweetness and antioxidants from the berries are provided by this easy and delicious treat.

6. Frozen Fruit Sorbet: Puree frozen fruits such as mangoes, pineapples, and peaches until smooth and creamy. The sweetness comes from the natural sugars in the fruits, and the texture is comparable to sorbet. Enjoy this guilt-free frozen delight as a light dessert.

Healthy Twist on Classic Desserts

Frozen treats may be enjoyed guilt-free by choosing healthier options that deliver wonderful tastes and pleasant textures while keeping nutritional value in mind. When compared to standard selections, these guilt-free frozen delights have fewer added sugars, harmful fats, and calories. Here's an explanation of guilt-free frozen treats, along with some examples:

1. Frozen Fruit Popsicles: Use pureed or blended fruits to make your own popsicles. Simply purée your favorite fruits, such as berries, mangoes, or watermelon, then pour into popsicle molds. If desired, add additional chopped fruits for texture. These handmade fruit popsicles are light, refreshing, and high in vitamins and fiber.

2. Greek Yogurt Parfait Popsicles: Create layers of Greek yogurt and fresh fruits in popsicle molds. Use plain Greek yogurt or lightly sweetened options. The Greek yogurt provides protein and creaminess, while the fruits add natural sweetness and vibrant colors. This frozen treat offers a balance of nutrients and a satisfying taste.

3. Banana "Nice" Cream: Slice ripe bananas and freeze them. Blend the frozen banana slices in a food processor or blender until smooth and creamy. You can enjoy the banana "nice" cream as is or customize it by adding a variety of mix-ins like cocoa powder, peanut butter, berries, or nuts. This guilt-free treat mimics the texture of ice cream without the added sugars or dairy.

4. Frozen Yogurt Bites: Place spoonfuls of flavored Greek yogurt on a parchment-lined baking sheet and freeze until solid. These bite-sized delights have the creamy feel of frozen yogurt and may be personalized with additional fruits, nuts, or a drizzle of dark chocolate for more taste and texture.

5. Frozen Berries with Whipped Cream: Freeze a combination of fresh berries, such as strawberries, blueberries, or raspberries. Serve with a spoonful of unsweetened coconut cream or Greek yogurt whipped cream. Natural sweetness and antioxidants from the berries are provided by this easy and delicious treat.

6. Frozen Fruit Sorbet: Puree frozen fruits such as mangoes, pineapples, and peaches until smooth and creamy. The sweetness comes from the natural sugars in the fruits, and the texture is comparable to sorbet. Enjoy this guilt-free frozen delight as a light dessert.

CHAPTER TEN

WEEK 1: KICKSTART YOUR NOOM JOURNEY

Daily Meal Plans and Recipes

Dinner Plan:

Breakfast: Omelette with Spinach and Mushrooms

Snack: Berries in Greek Yogurt

Lunch:

Quinoa Salad with Grilled Chicken

Snacks:

Carrot Sticks with Hummus as a Snack

Dinner:

Baked Salmon with Roasted Vegetables

Snack:

Almond Butter Apple Slices

Let's begin with the recipes:

Spinach and Mushroom Omelette:

Ingredients:

- 2 large eggs

- 12 cups thinly sliced mushrooms
- 1 cup chopped fresh spinach
- Season with salt and pepper to taste.
- Spray cooking oil or olive oil on the pan.

Instructions:

1. Whisk the eggs in a mixing bowl until well mixed. Season to taste with salt and pepper.

2. Heat a nonstick skillet with cooking spray or olive oil over medium heat.

3. Cook for a few minutes, or until the mushrooms are softened, in the skillet.

4. Cook the spinach in the skillet until it has wilted.

5. Pour the beaten eggs into the skillet, taking care to coat the vegetables evenly.

6. Cook for a few minutes more, or until the omelette is set. Gently fold the omelette in half.

7. Transfer to a serving dish and serve right away.

Greek yogurt with berries:

Ingredients:

- 1/2 pound of plain Greek yogurt (Berry Greek Yogurt)

- 1/4 cups of blueberries, raspberries, and strawberries
- Optional: 1 tablespoon honey or maple syrup

Instructions:

1. Scoop the Greek yogurt into a bowl.

2. Garnish with mixed berries.

3. If preferred, drizzle with honey or maple syrup.

4.Gently combine and serve.

Grilled Chicken Quinoa Salad:

Ingredients:

- 1/2 cups cooked quinoa
- 4 ounces sliced grilled chicken breast
- 1 cup mixed salad leaves
- 12 cups of halved cherry tomatoes
- 14 cups of sliced cucumber
- 2 tbsp. crumbled feta cheese
- 2 tbsp balsamic vinaigrette dressing

Instructions:

1. Toss together the cooked quinoa, mixed salad greens, cherry tomatoes, and cucumber in a large mixing basin.

2. Arrange the grilled chicken slices on top.

3. Toss the salad with the balsamic vinaigrette dressing to coat.

4. Top with crumbled feta cheese.

5. Serve right away.

Hummus on Carrot Sticks:

Ingredients:

- 2 medium peeled and sliced carrot sticks
- 1/4 cups of hummus

Instructions:

1. Wash and peel the carrots before cutting them into sticks.

2. To serve, dip the carrot sticks in hummus.

Salmon Baked with Roasted Vegetables:

Ingredients:

- 4 ounces of salmon fillet
- 1 cup chopped mixed veggies (broccoli, bell peppers, and zucchini)
- 1 teaspoon olive oil
- Season with salt and pepper to taste.
- Serve with lemon wedges.

Instructions:

1. Preheat the oven to 400 degrees Fahrenheit (200 degrees Celsius).

2. Line a baking sheet with parchment paper and place the salmon fillet on it.

3. In a separate bowl, toss the mixed veggies with olive oil, salt, and pepper.

4. Arrange the seasoned veggies on the baking sheet around the fish.

5. Bake for 15–20 minutes, or until the salmon is well cooked and the veggies are soft.

6. Serve the fish and veggies with lemon wedges for squeezing.

Almond Butter Apple Slices:

Ingredients:

- 1 medium sliced apple
- 2 teaspoons almond butter

Instructions:

1. Clean and cut the apple.

2. Toss the apple slices with the almond butter and serve

Tips for Meal Prepping and Batch Cooking

1. Plan Your Meals: Begin by making a weekly food plan. Take into account your nutritional requirements, dietary preferences, and any special goals you have in mind. Choose balanced dishes that include a range of veggies, lean meats, whole grains, and healthy fats.

2. Create a Grocery List: Once you've decided on a meal plan, make a grocery list of all the ingredients you'll need. This ensures that you have everything you need and reduces the need for last-minute food shop runs. To avoid impulsive purchases, stick to your shopping list.

3. Select Batch Cooking-Friendly Recipes: Look for recipes that can be easily scaled up and are batch-ready. Soups, stews, casseroles, and roasted vegetables are excellent choices since they can be cooked in bulk and saved for later use.

4. Schedule Prep Time: Set aside a set day or time during the week for meal planning and bulk preparation. This may be a weekend day or an evening with a few hours to kill. Use this time to prepare veggies, cereals, marinade meats, and put together meals.

5. Cook in Bulk: Make larger batches of your favorite dishes. You'll have leftovers for future dinners this way. Invest in freezer-safe food storage containers with distinct sections for various food products.

6. Portion Control: To make it easy to grab and go, divide your cooked meals into separate pieces. This aids in portion management and ensures you have meals ready to consume throughout the week. Label and date your containers to make them easier to identify.

7. Storage and Freezing: Depending on the shelf life of your prepared meals, keep them in the refrigerator or freezer. To keep food fresh and avoid freezer burn, use airtight containers or freezer bags. Keep track of expiration dates in order to consume meals with shorter shelf life first.

8. range and Flexibility: To avoid boredom, prepare a range of meals and snacks. Incorporate a variety of flavors, textures, and cuisines into your food plan. You may also prepare adaptable items like as roasted vegetables, cooked meats, or cooked grains that can be combined to make a variety of meals throughout the week.

9. Prepare nutritious Snacks: Don't forget to prepare nutritious snacks. For quick and nutritious snacks on the run, cut up fruits and veggies, divide out nuts or seeds, and make homemade energy balls or granola bars.

10. Food Safety and Hygiene: Pay attention to food safety measures when preparing meals. To avoid foodborne infections, wash your hands often, keep raw meats away from other components, and adhere to correct cooking temperatures and storage requirements.

CHAPTER ELEVEN

SUSTAINING HEALTHY HABITS

Daily Meal Plans and Recipes

Dinner Plan:

Breakfast:

Scrambled Eggs with Vegetables

Snack:

Berries in Greek Yogurt

Lunch:

Salad with Quinoa and Chickpeas

Snack:

Carrot Sticks with Hummus

Dinner:

Chicken grilled with roasted vegetables

Snack:

Almond Butter Apple Slices

Let's get started with the recipes:

Vegetable Scrambled Eggs:

Ingredients:

- 2 medium eggs
- 1/2 cup diced mixed veggies (such as bell peppers, spinach, and onions)
- To taste salt and pepper
- Cooking spray or olive oil for the pan

Instructions:

1. In a mixing basin, whisk the eggs until completely combined. Season with salt and pepper to taste.

2. Coat a nonstick pan with cooking spray or sprinkle with olive oil over medium heat.

3. Add the diced mixed veggies to the skillet and cook for a few minutes, or until softened.

4. Pour the beaten eggs into the skillet, being sure to evenly coat the veggies.

5. Cook, stirring gently, for a few minutes, or until the eggs are scrambled and cooked to your preference.

6. Transfer to a dish and serve immediately.

Berries in Greek Yogurt

Ingredients:

- 1/2 pound of plain Greek yogurt

- 1/4 cups mixed berries (blueberries, raspberries, and strawberries)
- Optional: 1 tablespoon honey or maple syrup

Instructions:

1. Scoop the Greek yogurt into a bowl.

2. Garnish with mixed berries.

3. If preferred, drizzle with honey or maple syrup.

4. Gently combine and serve.

Salad with Quinoa and Chickpeas:

Ingredients:

- 1/2 cups cooked quinoa
- 1/2 cups drained and washed canned chickpeas
- 1 cup salad greens, mixed
- 1/2 cups diced cucumber
- 1/4 cups of halved cherry tomatoes
- 2 teaspoons lemon juice
- 1 tablespoon olive oil
- season with salt and pepper to taste.

Instructions:

1. Toss together the cooked quinoa, chickpeas, mixed

salad greens, cucumber, and cherry tomatoes in a large mixing bowl.

2. To make the dressing, mix together the lemon juice, olive oil, salt, and pepper in a separate small bowl.
3. Toss the salad with the dressing to cover all of the ingredients.
4. Serve immediately or store in the refrigerator until ready to eat.

Hummus on Carrot Sticks:

Ingredients:

- 2 medium peeled and sliced carrot sticks
- 1/4 cups of hummus

Instructions:

1. Wash and peel the carrots before cutting them into sticks.
2. To serve, dip the carrot sticks in hummus.

Grilled Chicken and Roasted Vegetables:

Ingredients:

- 4 ounces boneless, skinless chicken breast
- 1 cup chopped mixed veggies (such as broccoli, bell peppers, and zucchini)

- 1 teaspoon olive oil
- Season with salt and pepper to taste
- Serve with lemon wedges.

Instructions:

1. Preheat the grill (or grill pan) over medium-high heat.

2. Season both sides of the chicken breast with salt and pepper.

3. Grill the chicken for 6–8 minutes per side, or until done.

4. Toss the mixed veggies with olive oil, salt, and pepper in a separate bowl.

5. Roast the veggies for 15–20 minutes, or until soft, in a preheated oven at 400°F (200°C).

6. Serve the grilled chicken with the roasted veggies and lemon juice.

Almond Butter Apple Slices:

Ingredients:

- 1 medium sliced apple
- 2 teaspoons almond butter

Instructions:

1. Wash and thinly slice the apple.

2. Toss the apple slices with the almond butter and serve.

How to Maintain Long-term Success

Long-term success in your health and wellness journey needs consistency, dedication, and a well-balanced approach. Here are some pointers to help you keep your momentum and achieve long-term results:

1. Establish Realistic objectives: Establish objectives that are precise, measurable, attainable, relevant, and time-bound (SMART goals). Larger objectives can be broken down into smaller milestones to help you stay motivated and measure your progress.

2. Concentrate on Long-Term improvements: Rather than depending on short-term solutions or fad diets, concentrate on achieving long-term lifestyle improvements. Incorporate healthy habits, such as mindful eating, frequent physical activity, and stress management strategies, gradually into your daily routine.

3. Create a Support Network: Surround yourself with a supportive network of friends, family, or like-minded people with similar aspirations. During difficult times, they may offer support, accountability, and advice.

4. Practice Mindful Eating: Practice mindful eating by observing your body's hunger and fullness cues, eating gently, and appreciating each mouthful. Rather than focusing entirely on calorie tracking, focus on consuming nutrient-dense meals that feed your body.

5. Maintain an Active Lifestyle: Engage in enjoyable physical activities on a regular basis. Find activities that you enjoy, such as walking, swimming, cycling, yoga, or strength training. To enhance general fitness and muscular mass, combine aerobic activity, strength training, and flexibility exercises.

6. Honor Non-Scale Victories: Honor accomplishments that go beyond the numbers on the scale. Recognize and recognize increases in energy levels, mood, sleep quality, strength, or self-confidence. These small wins can serve as strong motivators for long-term success.

7. Prioritize Self-Care Activities: Set aside time for self-care activities that help decrease stress, promote relaxation, and improve general well-being. This might include activities such as meditation, writing, spending time in nature, getting enough sleep, or participating in hobbies that you like.

8. Regularly Assess and Adjust: Reassess your objectives, methods, and progress on a regular basis. Be willing to change your strategy when your requirements and tastes change. Maintain flexibility and adaptability, since long-term success frequently necessitates changing and improving your strategy over time.

9. Maintain a good Attitude: Maintain a good attitude by focusing on self-compassion and self-acceptance. Negative self-talk and obsessing over setbacks should be avoided. Accept progress rather than perfection, and see any setbacks as learning opportunities rather than failures.

CHAPTER TWELVE

BEYOND THE 14-DAY PLAN: CUSTOMIZING YOUR NOOM DIET

Adapting the Noom Diet to Your Lifestyle

1. Make Gradual Changes: Rather than making big changes all at once, begin by gradually implementing Noom concepts into your lifestyle. Concentrate on one component at a time, such as boosting your vegetable intake or lowering your intake of added sugars. Build on these improvements gradually over time for long-term success.

2. Portion management: To help regulate portion sizes, practice portion management by utilizing smaller dishes and bowls. To construct balanced meals, use visual clues such as filling half your plate with veggies, one-fourth with lean protein, and one-fourth with nutritious grains.

3. Experiment with Recipes: Discover new recipes that adhere to the Noom Diet guidelines. Look for meals that are tasty and use whole, unadulterated foods. Experiment with different spices, herbs, and culinary techniques to spice up your dishes.

4. Meal Planning: Plan and prepare your meals ahead of time to ensure you have nutritious selections on hand. Spend time each week preparing ingredients or even entire meals to make healthy eating more accessible and achievable.

5. Choose Nutrient-Dense Snacks: Choose nutrient-dense snacks that fulfill your appetite while adhering to Noom's guidelines. Whole fruits, raw veggies with hummus, Greek yogurt with berries, or homemade trail mix with nuts and seeds are all good choices.

6. Mindful Eating: Slow down, appreciate each meal, and pay attention to your body's hunger and fullness signs to practice mindful eating. Avoid distractions such as watching TV or using technological gadgets when eating and instead concentrate on the sensory experience of your food.

7. Stay Hydrated: Drink lots of water throughout the day to stay hydrated. Water can help you lose weight, improve digestion, and stay energized. To enhance flavor, add fresh fruits, herbs, or a splash of citrus juice to your water.

8. Find Physical Activities You Love: Include physical activities in your regimen that you actually love. Choose things that keep you engaged and make exercise feel more like a pleasure than a chore, whether it's dancing, hiking, cycling, or taking dance lessons.

9. Personalize Noom's Color System: Make Noom's Color System work for you by customizing it to your tastes. Identify your favorite meals and place them in the proper color categories. This way, you can plan meals and snacks around your favorite foods. while still following the Noom principles.

Incorporating Flexibility and Moderation

Incorporating flexibility and moderation into your lifestyle can have a number of positive effects on your overall well-being. Here are some significant benefits of embracing flexibility and moderation in your eating and lifestyle habits:

1. Sustainable living: Moderation and flexibility foster sustainable living. Allowing yourself freedom in your food choices and embracing moderation creates a balanced eating style that can be maintained in the long run. It lowers the chances of feeling deprived or limited, making it simpler to maintain good behaviors over time.

112

2. Improved Psychological Well-Being: Adopting a flexible and reasonable approach fosters a healthy relationship with food and your body. It lessens the proclivity for tight regulations, guilt, or bad feelings related to eating. This encourages a good attitude, enhanced self-acceptance, and general psychological well-being.

3. Freedom from Food Obsession: Embracing flexibility and moderation frees you from worrying over food choices or feeling compelled to adhere to stringent dietary guidelines. It enables more intuitive and attentive eating, allowing you to heed your body's demands and urges while still making nutritional choices.

4. Increased Nutritional Variety: Flexibility and moderation promote a varied and well-balanced diet. You may receive a wide range of nutrients, vitamins, and minerals from diverse food sources by allowing yourself to enjoy a variety of meals in moderation. This helps to maintain total nutritional balance and good health.

5. Weight control: Adopting a flexible and moderate approach can help with weight control. It aids in the prevention of the vicious cycle of excessive dieting followed by overindulgence. You can maintain a healthy weight range without resorting to restrictive diets or severe measures by making balanced food choices and exercising portion management.

6. Social pleasure: Including flexibility and moderation provides for greater pleasure at social events and occasions. You may attend social gatherings, eat meals with friends and family, and treat yourself on occasion without feeling alienated or separated from your social group.

7. Less Deprivation: Flexibility and moderation reduce the sensation of deprivation that is typically linked with tight diets. Allowing yourself to consume modest quantities of your favorite foods or indulge on occasion can help fulfill cravings and reduce feelings of restriction, leading to a more pleasant and sustainable eating pattern.

8. Increased Adherence to Healthy Behaviors: Flexibility and moderation make it simpler to maintain healthy behaviors over time. Allowing oneself flexibility allows you to adjust to diverse settings, travel, and unforeseen occurrences without becoming disheartened. It assists you in navigating life's obstacles while leading a healthy lifestyle.

Troubleshooting and Managing Plateaus

The occurrence of plateaus in your health and wellness journey is typical. Plateaus are moments when you may not notice any progress toward your weight reduction or fitness objectives. However, with the correct troubleshooting methods, you may overcome plateaus and keep moving forward toward your goals. Here are some pointers for dealing with plateaus:

1. Reevaluate Your objectives: Take some time to review your objectives to verify they are still relevant to your current requirements and aspirations. Are they reachable and realistic? If your objectives are no longer helping you or if you have already attained them, you may need to revise them.

2. Track Your Food and Exercise: Go over your food and exercise diaries to ensure you're documenting your intake and activity levels correctly. Inconsistencies in tracking can sometimes result from complacency or forgetfulness, which can stymie development. Consider keeping a food journal or using a monitoring app to keep track of your consumption and exercise.

3. Examine Portion Sizes: Examine your portion sizes to ensure that you're practicing portion control properly. It's easy to lose track of portion amounts over time, which might contribute to plateaus. To guarantee you're eating the right amount, use measuring cups or a food scale.

4. Vary Your training program: Plateaus can arise when your body becomes acclimated to a specific training program. Include new workouts, various intensities, or alternative hobbies to add diversity and push your body. This keeps your body from adjusting and encourages continual improvement.

5. Adjust Your Caloric Intake: If you have been following a certain calorie target, reconsider your caloric requirements. Your calorie needs may fluctuate as you lose weight or make progress. Consult a qualified dietitian or healthcare practitioner to see whether your calorie intake needs to be adjusted.

6. Examine Your Macronutrient Distribution: Examine your macronutrient distribution to ensure you're receiving the right combination of carbs, protein, and healthy fats. Adjusting your macronutrient ratios might occasionally help you break through plateaus and accelerate your development.

7. Examine Your Sleep and Stress Levels: Sleep deprivation and chronic stress can have an impact on your metabolism and general well-being, perhaps contributing to plateaus. Prioritize proper sleep and seek out appropriate stress-management approaches, such as relaxation techniques, exercising, or engaging in fun hobbies.

8. Concentrate on Non-Scale Victories: Stop relying entirely on the scale. Non-scale triumphs, such as more energy, higher fitness, better sleep, or beneficial changes in body composition, should be celebrated. These accomplishments might help you stay motivated and keep a positive attitude.

9. Seek Support and Accountability: Consider reaching out to a support system or working with a healthcare practitioner, certified dietitian, or personal trainer. Based on your individual circumstances, they can provide direction, accountability, and assistance in troubleshooting plateaus.

10. Be Patient and persistent. Recognize that plateaus are a natural part of the journey and that progress is not

always linear. Maintain patience, consistency, and faith in the process. Plateaus are transient and may be surmounted with time and persistence.

CONCLUSION

In conclusion, the "Noom Diet Cookbook and Meal Plan" offers a thorough guide to assist you in embarking on a path toward a healthy lifestyle. The Noom Diet, with its emphasis on psychology, behavior modification, and long-term habits, provides a novel approach to reaching and sustaining weight reduction and wellness objectives.

We have studied the concept and principles of the Noom Diet throughout this book, learning how it works, the advantages it provides, and practical techniques for incorporating it into your everyday life. The Noom Diet promotes a balanced and flexible approach to nutrition by stressing portion management, nutrient-dense foods, and mindful eating.

We've spoken about how important it is to create objectives, make specific strategies, and keep track of your progress. You can overcome obstacles, stay motivated, and build good habits that will lead to long-term success if you follow the advice presented.

The Noom Color System has been described, allowing you to make more educated food selections and maintain a healthy diet balance. The Noom Diet Cookbook and Meal Plan includes a wide choice of delectable dishes to keep you content and fed, from nutrient-dense dinners and protein-packed treats to savory salads and innovative snacks.

We've also talked about the importance of portion management, filling your pantry for success, and the important equipment and gadgets that will help you with your culinary ventures. In addition, we have included recommendations for healthy grocery shopping, allowing you to make informed decisions while you navigate the aisles.

You may enjoy a variety of nourishing and tasty meals while promoting weight reduction, improved general health, and greater well-being by implementing the Noom Diet concepts into your lifestyle. This method is based on flexibility, moderation, and a balanced mentality, allowing you to handle social settings while still enjoying your favorite meals without feeling guilty or deprived.

As you continue on this road, keep in mind that long-term success necessitates patience, perseverance, and an optimistic attitude. It is critical to listen to your body, prioritize self-care, and seek help when necessary. With the "Noom Diet Cookbook and Meal Plan" as your guide, you may adopt a healthy lifestyle and achieve long-term benefits.

Now that you've mastered the Noom Diet concept, meal planning, and a variety of dishes, it's time to go on your personal wellness journey. Adopt the Noom Diet principles, make conscious decisions, and enjoy the tasty and nutritious meals that will fuel your body and boost your well-being. Here's to a happy, healthier you!

Printed in Great Britain
by Amazon

43970664R00069